Safari

Marc Maurer
Editor

Large Type Edition

A KERNEL BOOK
published by
NATIONAL FEDERATION OF THE BLIND

TABLE OF CONTENTS

EDITOR'S INTRODUCTION

Safari suggests Africa, mystery, the jungle, danger. What is dangerous for a blind person? Getting lost? Bumping into something? Being bitten by a scorpion in the Grand Canyon? These could all be serious, but more serious still is the failure by blind people and their friends to understand our potential. Much worse than getting lost is never to attempt the safari at all.

Hence the title for the newest volume in our Kernel Book series, *Safari*. It means a journey of high adventure—shared with others, with you. In the decade since the beginning of the Kernel Book series, we who are blind and you who have become our friends have truly shared a journey—a journey which in its own way is as exciting and demanding and adventurous as any safari through the African jungle.

We have traveled together through the whole range of human emotions—from the depths of despair which can and often does accompany blindness to the exultation of acceptance, achievement, and accomplishment. And you have been with us every step of the way. In story after story our lives have unfolded, and you have shared our heartaches and our triumphs.

In the present volume we continue together on safari. You will meet friends of mine who I hope will become your friends, too. They are the ordinary blind men and women who make up the National Federation of the Blind—individuals whose daily lives give form and substance to our belief that blindness need not be the terrible tragedy it is almost universally assumed to be.

Among these new friends you will find a blind tax attorney who on a real-life safari negotiates with an African chieftain; a blind scoutmaster who leads a rim-to-rim-to-rim

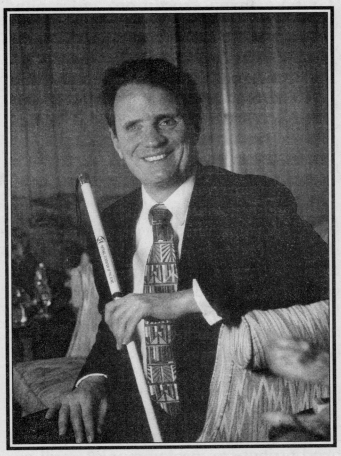

Marc Maurer, President
National Federation of the Blind

Grand Canyon expedition; and a blind father who is told that his twelve-year-old daughter must act as "a responsible adult" to care for him.

It is impossible to over-emphasize the central role our sighted friends play in our struggle to deal with the difficulties posed by blindness. We often say that our real problems come not from the lack of eyesight itself, but from what all of us (blind and sighted alike) have grown up thinking about blindness. The notions of darkness and terror and despair that dominate the prevailing image of blindness need have no part in our lives as we live them on a daily basis. But you must help us put those false images to rest.

Only when blind people come to be seen as ordinary human beings—as friends, neighbors, and coworkers with something to contribute to the community—will our safari come to its end.

The essence of our message is simple. We need training. We need opportunity. We need understanding. Our stories go to the very heart of blindness, trying to show our readers what it's really like to be blind—and, for that matter, what it isn't like.

I hope you will enjoy this 21st Kernel Book and that you will continue on safari with us for years to come. The journey is exciting, and with the tens of thousands of friends we have made through the Kernel Books accompanying us, the eventual successful outcome is assured.

Marc Maurer
Baltimore, Maryland
2001

WHY LARGE TYPE?

The type size used in this book is 14 point for two important reasons: One, because typesetting of 14 point or larger complies with federal standards for the printing of materials for visually impaired readers, and we want to show you what type size is helpful for people with limited sight.

The second reason is that many of our friends and supporters have asked us to print our paperback books in 14-point type so they too can easily read them. Many people with limited sight do not use Braille. We hope that by printing this book in a larger type than customary, many more people will be able to benefit from it.

THE SUNSET, THE GIRLFRIEND, AND THE MOTORCYCLE

by Marc Maurer

I have been blind all my life, and I have never "seen" a sunset. This has troubled my mind occasionally—but not very much. For all of my adult life I have been a member of the National Federation of the Blind, and I have served as its President for fifteen years. One of the things that we in the Federation often say is that the ordinary blind person is very much like the ordinary sighted person except for the inability to see. We share the hopes and dreams of our sighted colleagues, and we have many of the same objectives, beliefs, and fears.

If you take an average group of blind people, it will have members who are as energetic, as intelligent, as filled with fun, and as inspiring as the average group of sighted people. It will also contain people who are as idiotic, as lazy, and as dull.

Why do I bring this up? A number of people who think they know a lot about blindness keep telling us that blindness makes us fundamentally different from other people, but we don't believe it. Nevertheless, it is apparent that in certain respects blind people are indeed different from the sighted—not dramatically or fundamentally different, but different. Part of it has to do with expectations.

In discussing the difference between the blind and the sighted one phenomenon frequently raised is the sunset. The colors, the quality of light, the interaction between day and night, the grandeur of the experience, and the symbolism are (it is often believed) experiences the blind cannot have. When I began to ponder the question of how blind people are different from the sighted, I thought about the sunset. I had been told that a picture of a sunset is indistinguishable from a picture of a sunrise—that the visual image is identical. Even though the two events are dramatically different, they look the same if the only sets of characteristics are those connected directly with the sun itself. A sunset is not just a visual image.

When I asked some of my friends to describe a sunset, I discovered that one of my longtime sighted colleagues had never really looked at one. She found it fascinating to observe the pattern of light and shadow, the differing shades of refracted illumination, and the altering images created in the landscape.

The sunset described to me occurred as we were standing at the edge of the sea. The sun approaching the horizon made a path across the water. The rays of the setting disc made a visual impression like trumpets that would open a major event. The shade of reflected light from the water was pink across the horizon. Clouds in the sky between us and the sun reflected the light and caused an impression of a fight between the sun and the clouds. The display of color contained beauty and drama which lasted between twenty minutes and half an hour.

Because I had anticipated asking questions about the sunset, I had earlier sat in my own backyard on a spring evening recording my own impressions of this phenomenon without any visual description.

Over a period of about forty-five minutes, the warmth of the sunshine, which I could feel on my face, diminished and disappeared. Birds which had been singing in the trees became silent, but the owls began to call. Later during the year, I would have expected the insects to commence a chorus of night sounds, but this sunset was early in the spring before the insects had developed sufficiently to add their notes.

However, the evening breeze began to sigh gently in the trees, and the leaves on the ground were making their dry, rattling, scurrying noises. In addition, there were the barks of distant dogs and the occasional sound of traffic a long way off. The overwhelming impression was one of peace and calm although a whole panorama of sound—gentle sound—accompanied the coming of night. My impression of a sunset is less dramatic than the description I was given, but the calmness and peace contain a beauty of their own.

Although I have never observed a sunset in precisely the same way that my sighted colleagues have done it, I have an impression of the experience. I suspect that my notion of a sunset takes at least a little of its spirit from the poems I have read along with the memory of sitting with friends beside a campfire on a fall evening, and I am sure there are a hundred other factors.

Do blind people enjoy the sunset more or less than the sighted? It depends, it seems to me, on the people involved. Some care; some don't. When I was having the sunset described to me, there were three sighted people giving me a blow-by-blow narrative. One of these was a trained observer. She had been responsible for describing many visual images to blind people. Her description was filled with detail.

However, a different sighted person simply said that the color was magnificent. It may have been that he did not have either the interest or the training to observe individual details, though he is generally articulate. Perhaps, he did not see as much in the sunset as my other colleague. Which leads to the reflection that observation is not only a matter of vision—it requires training and the willingness to notice pattern and detail.

Sometimes the difference between the blind and the sighted is more complicated than the sunset, but it still involves expectations. As the President of the National Federation of the Blind, I am often asked to solve unusual questions. At a recent meeting of blind people within the National Federation of the Blind, I was asked by a blind man how he should go about finding a girlfriend. I have experience with this problem, and I did my best to answer the question.

It is perhaps an obvious oversimplification that girlfriends must be discovered where they are. Some people look in bars or nightclubs, but I have had poor success in such places, so I do not recommend this.

The techniques necessarily used by the blind for interacting with members of the opposite sex are somewhat restricted in the nightclub setting. To get to know somebody else, it is usually necessary to have at least a little conversation. Some nightclubs are so noisy that hearing the dulcet tones of a companion is virtually impossible.

Consequently, I look for company in other places, where conversation is much more likely. One of the best locations to become friendly with others is at church. School is good, and some find close friends at work. However, church is a place with a wide range of human beings who are at least trying to live decent lives.

Go to church, I told the blind man, and do not simply show up for Sunday service, but for other events as well. Volunteers are limited, and anybody who comes for activities in the church and tries to lend a hand will be highly regarded and gladly accepted. In the course of time it will be possible to talk with other members of the congregation, and friendships may be made. With a little effort a friendship with a young lady may progress. She may be persuaded to become a girlfriend.

When I was much younger, before I became a married man, I dated girls myself. Often I double-dated with a buddy I befriended at college. He was a good guy, and he owned a car, which was handy for me. We enjoyed working on his automobile together at times when we were not dating, and we became good friends.

One evening we had our girlfriends with us at his house. My buddy said that another friend of his had parked his Harley-Davidson motorcycle in the backyard. He said that his friend would not mind if we borrowed it. The Harley had a sidecar attached. The battery on the motorcycle was dead, so we had to kick start the machine. At the time, I weighed about one hundred twenty-five pounds, and my buddy was not much heavier. We both tried to get some life into the cycle, but we failed.

We decided that the only way to start the cycle was to push it and pop the clutch. I got on one side and my buddy on the other. We began to run—actually it was more like a slow lumber—and we popped the clutch. The motorcycle skidded to a stop without making a sound.

What to do? My buddy drove a four-on-the-floor, stick-shift Ford. Neither of the girls knew how to drive a stick. My buddy said that we would need to push the motorcycle with the Ford. I volunteered to drive.

My buddy and his girlfriend took seats—he on the motorcycle and she in the sidecar. I started the Ford and put it in gear. Very gently, I began to push the motorcycle. Within a few seconds it started, and off they went. My girlfriend told me to stop the car. She was not prepared to ride, she said.

Misadventures sometimes occurred on my dates. I remember one evening in the spring when I was walking with my girlfriend down by the river. We came to an out-of-the-way footbridge, and we started across it. I learned, to my surprise, that part of the bridge had no railing.

As I was teetering on the edge about to fall off, my girlfriend grabbed me by the collar of my jacket. In those days I had not yet learned that it is of utmost importance for a blind person to carry a cane. I often tried to learn about new surroundings through the soles of my feet—a precarious and sometimes dangerous thing to do.

Although my girlfriend held tightly to my coat, it didn't stop me. My arms flew into the air and slid from the sleeves of my jacket;

and I fell into the river. Fortunately, I am a good swimmer, and the bridge was not a high one. I was able to return to it within a few seconds, completely drenched.

Most of my dates were the more customary kind—participation in school dances, visits to restaurants or ice cream parlors, travels to the movies or other entertainment, or sitting holding hands. To find a girlfriend a guy must demonstrate that he is interesting enough to attract a girl. This problem is essentially the same for the blind as it is for the sighted.

We in the National Federation of the Blind want to be a part of our community. We dream of a bright tomorrow for ourselves and for our sighted friends and neighbors, and we are prepared to work to make the dream come true.

Because we hope to work with you and play with you and build with you, we have often told you how much we are alike, but there are also the small differences—the differences that help to make us interesting. Even with these small differences, we can still enjoy a sunset, hope for an exciting date, or ride on a motorcycle.

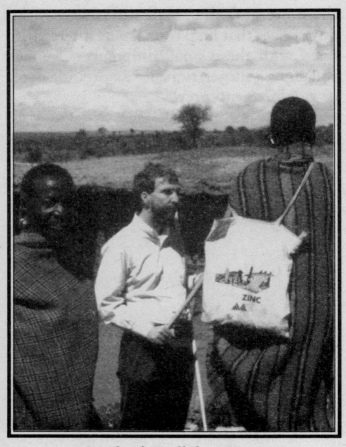

Michael Baillif in Kenya

SAFARI

by Michael Baillif

Seasoned Kernel Book readers will remember Michael Baillif as the fifteen-year-old who scrambled up onto the roof one balmy summer evening to write love poetry. Today Michael is a successful tax attorney. He was recently married, and he and his wife Lynn are busy settling into their first home in the historic Baltimore neighborhood known as Federal Hill. But here we meet him on safari in Africa, where in a thousand-year-old village, Michael reflects with insight and humor on today's realities. Here is what he has to say:

Our van had been bumping, thumping, and skidding over the nearly impassable road for what seemed like an eternity. Finally, we had reached our destination—a village of a tribe known as the Masai Mara located in the Serengeti plain in Kenya, Africa. As part of a family vacation, we had ventured to Kenya and spent the last several days traveling from Nairobi to Mount Kenya, and now to the Serengeti plain. As one of the final stops before beginning the interminable homeward trip to the United States, we had decided to seek out a village, which but for the malign influence of tourists like us, was functioning more or less as it had for thousands of years.

After digging out my cane from between the van seats, where it had become almost immovably wedged, I stepped out of the van and breathed a sigh of relief. It was almost my last. I inhaled a cloud of dust particles that sent me into a paroxysm of coughing. When I had recovered sufficiently, I asked our guide "What is all of that dust blowing around?" "Oh, that's dry camel dung." he said. "The villagers use it to plaster together their houses."

Attempting to breathe as shallowly as possible, I followed our group into the village. We were given a tour by one of the villagers who, with the aid of our guide, explained how the village operated and described a normal day in the life of a Masai Mara tribesman. He told us of how they cultivated maize and talked of occasional expeditions to hunt water-buck and gazelle.

We were even able to walk through one of the houses, a hut really, and watch as an elderly grandmother prepared the evening meal over an open fire. As we were observing this, the tribesman who had been showing us around approached one of my family members and asked if I was really blind. He shook his head sadly, and said "Can't see, too bad, too bad."

I wanted to explain that blindness really wasn't much of an issue for me because I had been lucky enough to acquire the attitudes and skills I needed to do pretty much whatever I wanted. But, given the language barrier, the best I could do was to point to my cane, make a dismissive gesture, and say "It's ok."

As we walked out of the hut, I reflected to myself that one can travel the world and be confronted with astonishingly consistent views regarding blindness. Be it at an American university, an English pub, or an African village, the odds are high that one will encounter the same types of attitudes about blindness. People tend to look upon blindness as awful and upon blind people as being sometimes worthless, sometimes admirable, and not uncommonly as being both at once.

Of course, the reality is much different. Blindness, like any other characteristic, is no more and no less than what we, and our larger society, make of it. Given good training of the kind provided by the National Federation of the Blind, positive attitudes, sufficient opportunities, and a community that doesn't get in the way, blindness really need not be a big deal.

But until these elements of equality become the norm, the social outlook, and occasional reality, will be that blindness is a terrible thing.

I was pondering how these attitudes regarding blindness could best be overcome when my musings were interrupted by the village chieftain who had been leading our tour. He offered to sell me an African war club, hand-carved out of a single piece of teakwood. It really was beautiful and packed a whollop that would knock the recipient into next Sunday. All of a sudden, at least superficially, he had apparently come to terms with my blindness and now was cheerfully endeavoring to sell me the same products that were being offered to others in the group.

I asked the price of the club. He quoted me a price of 250 shillings, but said that since I was his good friend, I could have it for 100 shillings. I told him that I would think about the deal and went to confer with other members of my group. As it turned out, someone else had purchased a similar club for 100 shillings as well.

I returned to the villager and asked, "If I'm your good friend, how come I don't get a better deal than those guys?" We negotiated some more, but he held firm at 100 shillings.

Finally admitting defeat, I agreed to purchase the war club at his price. In order to complete our transaction, all that remained was to calculate the exchange rate between Kenyan shillings and U.S. dollars. This task took a bit longer than expected, though, because my friend kept trying to shave a few cents off of the exchange rate to his benefit.

What he did not know is that by trade I am a tax attorney. While tax attorneys may possess innumerable shortcomings, one thing we can do is keep track of the money flowing into and out of our pockets.

As I left the Masai Mara village carrying my newly-acquired war club, I was quite pleased. The negotiations in general and my friend's attempted larceny in particular had made me feel good.

The very man who had pitied me and genuinely felt sorry for my fate was, only a few minutes later, prepared to treat me as the equal of any sighted person where our economic transaction was concerned. Once the villager realized that I had something he wanted, he saw me in a much different light from the person for whom only sorrow and pity had been appropriate.

Whether or not the villager's actual perceptions of blindness changed on the spot, I couldn't tell, but in a certain sense, I didn't necessarily care. What mattered to me more than what he might have thought about blindness was how he treated me as a blind person. Judging by that standard, I had been the recipient of equality safari-style.

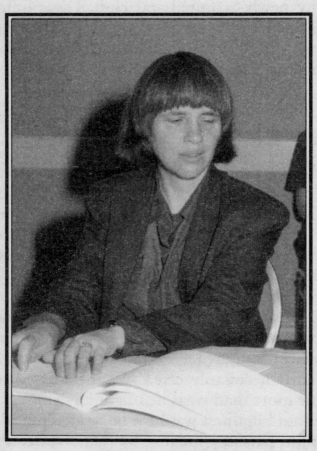

Peggy Elliott

SNAKES

by Peggy Elliott

Peggy Elliott is Second Vice President of the National Federation of the Blind, and her stories have appeared in many previous Kernel Books. There is really no way to describe her current offering except to say that it is delightful. Hope you enjoy it as much as I did. Here is what she has to say:

I have lived in this small Upper Midwestern town for most of my life, and my family has three generations of history here. I can show you where my grandparents used to live, the places in the community center where my locker was located when the building was a junior high, the site in the downtown park where the little merry-go-round with the horses used to twirl us. I feel I belong here.

As blind persons, we don't always feel we belong. We yearn to be part of our world, to help make the coffee or bring the cupcakes, to be appointed or elected, to be greeted as one of the crowd when we arrive. Many of our fellow citizens feel this same way about us, but others are unsure how to talk to us or lack confidence that we can do what others do. And, sometimes we blind people aren't sure of ourselves, either. We do want to belong, but can we?

I have used a white cane for thirty years now and, in my town, that means using the white cane in ice and snow for part of the year. Winter conditions are actually often easier to get around in when you use a white cane because the sidewalks and streets are lined with snow, providing an extra big cue to where you are. Sidewalks are tramped or shoveled, so there is an extra set of clues to find and follow when using the white cane. And, besides, I like cold weather or I wouldn't want to live here. But then please remember that I do belong here.

I walk to work every day. In winter, that often means walking while there is still undisturbed snow on the ground, a new layer of an inch or two over the trodden path along the sidewalk. I use my white cane, moving it from side to side in front of me as I walk along the sidewalk. That's just the way I walk. I never thought about the marks I was leaving until the day the neighbor started laughing.

I was walking south toward town when I heard a man approaching, laughing, and calling my name. I stopped to talk and found that he was a neighbor of mine, living north of us and heading back home from his morning walk. As we met, he continued to laugh and said, "Now I know what those are!"

I was enjoying his merriment but puzzled about what the "those" were about which he was laughing. "Those marks!" he said several times, still laughing.

My neighbor explained that he walks every day and, once the snow started, had noticed marks in the snow, marks like a snake moving purposefully down the sidewalk, weaving back and forth as it went. He couldn't figure out what the marks were until he saw me approaching. The motion of my cane back and forth told him what made the snakes in the snow.

My snakes in the snow belong there. They are my way of finding where I am and of keeping myself safe as I walk. And, for anybody in my town who has seen them, they tell the story: Peggy has been by here since the last snowfall. It's part of how I belong.

THE GRAND CANYON: FROM RIM TO RIM TO RIM

by Bruce A. Gardner

Bruce Gardner is a member of the National Federation of the Blind Board of Directors and President of the NFB of Arizona. He is the father of six and a leader in his community and his church. He has an extremely responsible job as an attorney. I have not the remotest idea how he finds time to do all the things he does, but one of them is participating with his sons in scouting activities.

Over the years Bruce has learned to be patient with those who think his blindness should keep him from being a top-notch scout. And his patience has paid off. After all, it's pretty hard not to believe in a man who can hike the Grand Canyon rim to rim to rim. Here is what he has to say:

For most of my adult life I have served in one capacity or another as a volunteer leader with the Boy Scouts of America. The last few years I have served as a scout troop committee chairman. Last summer I hiked the Grand Canyon with my son Bruce and the other Explorer Scouts (sixteen- to eighteen-year-old boys) from our troop. We hiked from the South Rim to the North Rim and back to the South Rim, which was approximately fifty miles. Unlike the other fifty-mile hikes I have taken, there is very little flat or level hiking in the Canyon.

We camped in the National Forest at the top of the South Rim the first night. Early the next morning we put on our backpacks containing our sleeping bags, camp stoves, food, water, and other gear and headed down the Canyon. The sheer cliffs and scenic vistas were simply breathtaking.

The first leg of the trail was about seven or eight miles to the Colorado River at the bottom of the Canyon, which is more than

ten or eleven miles away as the crow flies. It seemed strange to realize that at the bottom of the Canyon we had hiked through a blazing hot desert, while at the rim of the Canyon we were enjoying the cool pines.

After lunch we marched back down the North Rim to the bottom of the Canyon, and across the desert floor back to the Colorado River, where we cooked dinner and bedded down for the night. All told, we had put in about twenty-one or twenty-two miles that day. Early the next morning we cooked breakfast, packed up our gear, strapped on our backpacks, and started up the ten-mile trail back to the top of the South Rim.

By the time I reached the top of the South Rim, it was clear that my get-up-and-go had got up and went—I was tired. The last 4.5 miles up the Bright Angel Trail is called the wall because it is nonstop switchbacks. It seemed a little like walking up a four-and-a-half-mile staircase.

The two walking sticks I made from agave wood (a desert plant commonly known as century plant) were as helpful for taking the strain off my knees as they were as white canes. At the bottom of the Canyon we had been hoping for some cloud cover or rain, but we did not get much that day until we were about a half mile from the top. At that point a little thundercloud rolled in and drenched us. It felt good at first, but when we crested the Rim, we were soon chilled.

Although we were cold, wet, and exhausted, it was a thrill to reach the top. The entire trip was tremendous. As we sat under some shelter to rest and wait for the rain to stop, we looked out over the Canyon. I could not help comparing this scouting adventure with others I had experienced. This trip had been different.

As we planned for this hike, about half of the fifteen scouts wanted to hike to the bottom of the Canyon, spend a day or so, and then hike out, while the other half (the high school athletes) began challenging each other to hike rim to rim to rim. Of the four adult leaders hiking with the fifteen young men, I was the only adult who was interested in the extended trek. Because I had hiked the Grand Canyon twice before, once down and out in one day, and once backpacking from rim to rim, I had hoped some day to hike from rim to rim to rim.

We decided to divide into two groups, and I would serve as adult supervisor for the hardy boys. No one questioned my ability to hike or supervise the scouts, and no one suggested that someone would need to be assigned to take care of me. The fact that I was blind was never an issue.

Of course it had not always been that way. Once when I was a Boy Scout at junior leader training at summer camp, we were scheduled to go on a night hike. I had been a scout for about three years and had been on many hikes. In fact, I had earned the Eagle Scout award the previous year.

However, the leaders of the summer camp assumed that I would not be able to make the hike and did not want to take the risk of having a blind boy go on the night hike, so I was not allowed to go. The fact that I was an Eagle Scout, had earned the hiking merit badge, and had served as a guide for other Scout troops on a thirty-five-mile historic trail hike in Southern Utah made no difference. I was blind—that was all that mattered. Therefore I was not allowed to go on the hike.

It hurt to be denied the opportunity to go on the hike with the other scouts at the junior leader training. But at that time I had not yet heard of the National Federation of the Blind and did not know how to deal with others who treated me as if I were helpless.

As I said, this hike in the Grand Canyon was different. It was even different from hikes I had been on with these same boys as recently as four or five years earlier when I had spent the week with them at summer camp. During that week at camp we had gone on several short (three- to five-mile) hikes. One of the boys' fathers (a neighbor of mine) came up to camp for a couple of days and went on one of the hikes. He was shocked to learn that I was participating with the boys on all their activities. As we hiked that day, he took it upon himself to serve as my guardian and personal protector.

He walked in front of me along the trail feverishly trying to remove all the obstacles along the way. If there was a rock or log in the trail too big for him to move, he would attempt to grab me and physically maneuver me around it. Of course I did not put up with that, so he resorted to trying to walk backwards ahead of me so he could watch my every move and orally guide me through each obstacle.

The young scouts got quite a chuckle at the spectacle he made. Of course it would not do to get mad or become offended, so I patiently explained to him that this type of assistance was not necessary and that the white cane I was using told me where the obstacles were.

Gradually he relaxed a little so that by the end of the hike that day he had turned most of his attention to visiting with his son and only occasionally would he attempt to serve as my personal protector. Of course that evening around the campfire he could not stop talking about how wonderful I was.

Later that night I went to take a shower. The shower house was two or three campsites away. After I left our camp, this same neighbor turned to the other adults and asked, "Isn't someone going to go with him? He will get lost." The others in camp just shrugged their shoulders and told him I knew what I was doing.

When I did not return promptly, he began asking others returning from the showers if they had seen me. Because none of them had, he was convinced that I had gotten lost, and he suggested that a search party be formed to look for me. When I finally sauntered back into camp, my would-be protector was greatly relieved. He asked where I had been, and my casual reply seemed to dumbfound him.

I explained that on my way to the showers I had come across two very young scouts who were lost, scared, and in need of help. They had become separated from their scout troop while on a night compass course hike. When I found them, they had been wandering, hopelessly lost for nearly an hour. Their flashlights had grown dim, and the boys were obviously scared and worried about all the night sounds around them.

When they saw me, they simultaneously burst into nervous, excited chatter. They described their plight and asked me how to get to their campsite. When I explained that their camp was about a half mile away, they asked if I would take them there, and of course I did. Then I returned and took my shower.

All of this seemed to be beyond my neighbor's comprehension. I was blind. How could I possibly do a normal thing like help lost scouts find their way back to camp? Gradually, however, my neighbor has come to understand that blindness does not mean helplessness and that by using alternative techniques we who are blind can enjoy full and productive lives.

Well, as I said, the scout hike last summer in the Grand Canyon was a wonderful, exhilarating, exhausting adventure, and the fact that my blindness was never made an issue made it especially rewarding.

LET 'EM RIDE

by Curtis Chong

Curtis Chong was born and raised in Hawaii. He lived for many years in Minnesota, where he was employed as a senior level computer analyst with American Express. He now serves as Director of Technology for the National Federation of the Blind. Since he regards himself as a responsible adult, he was not pleased when the management of an amusement park wanted his twelve-year-old daughter to assume responsibility for him. Here is what he has to say:

Most people enjoy the thrills and adventure of an amusement park. As a person who has been blind from birth, my enjoyment of wild rides like the roller coaster, the octopus, the salt-and-pepper shaker, and other rides which fling you around in exciting and unpredictable ways is no less because of my inability to see. In fact, the thrill of the ride is heightened when we can't tell what is going to happen next. The fear, anticipation, and surprise are what make amusement park rides truly fun and enjoyable.

Throughout the course of my life, I have visited and enjoyed quite a few amusement parks. I have been to Disneyland in Anaheim, California, and Six Flags in Dallas, Texas. Rarely has anyone questioned my ability to ride, nor has anyone made a big deal about my blindness. Every once in a while, I will give my white cane to the ride operator, but for the most part, I ride the rides, experience the thrill, and have a terrific time--just like anybody else.

A few years ago, I had occasion to take my then twelve-year-old daughter Tina (who was and is fully sighted) and a group of friends to an amusement park in Minnesota called ValleyFair. I had every expectation

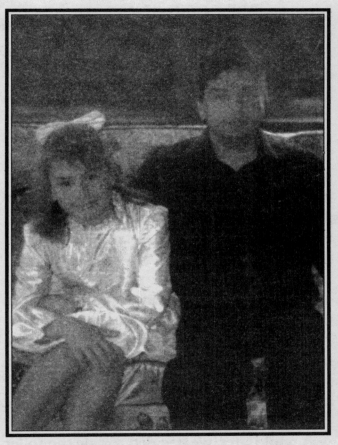

Curtis Chong and his daughter Tina

that we were all going to have a terrific time. After all, ValleyFair was reputed to be an excellent amusement park with the most exciting rides. I was sure to be flung, dropped, flipped, and otherwise thrown about, and I was looking forward to having a marvelous time.

My first intimation of trouble occurred at the entrance gate. The attendant, who made a point of speaking to my daughter instead of me, said, "You need to take him to Guest Relations so they can tell him what he can ride."

I asked politely if I was actually required to visit Guest Relations, and I was told that I was not. Therefore, I made some polite noises about visiting Guest Relations when I had time and went on my merry way. I should have heeded this warning.

A while later, we decided to ride the roller coaster. I went with Tina and a friend of hers, who was approximately her age, and stood in the line for this very popular ride. When we were about to board, the ride operator turned to my daughter and said, "He (meaning me) has to ride with you."

That simple statement was made with casual disregard of the fact that it was I, the adult, not Tina who was supposed to be in charge of the group. It spoke volumes about the ride operator's perception of blindness and the capabilities of blind people. Without meaning to, the operator (who probably had never met a competent blind person before) automatically assumed that I, the blind person, was being taken care of by the people around me who could see.

Tina was quite rightly annoyed. After all, she wanted to ride with her friend—not with her father. According to her way of thinking, I was quite capable of riding the roller coaster by myself. My years of active involvement in the National Federation of the Blind had taught me that blind people were just as capable as the sighted of living normal, productive, and enjoyable lives; and I had worked diligently to teach these ideas to Tina. To her, blindness was simply not anything to worry about. She had seen me do all kinds of things: operate a computer, make repairs around the house, work in an office, ride a bicycle, and so on. The thought that she would be required to sit with me, ostensibly to look after me, simply never occurred to her. And, based on my previously positive experiences with amusement parks, it never occurred to me either.

Frankly, I was surprised by what the ride operator was saying to my daughter and perhaps more than a little put out by the operator's blatant (if unintentional) dismissal of me as the leader of the group. After all, wasn't I the adult in charge of this little expedition? Who was supposed to be taking care of whom?

Tina and I tried to put up a fight, but the ride operator would have none of it. Either

Tina would sit with me or we would not ride. It was that simple. So, Tina had to sit with me. Neither she nor I was at all happy about how things were turning out.

I felt that, whether I liked it or not, the time had come to visit Guest Relations. I had to find out what the rules actually said. As it turned out, there were quite a few rules dealing with people with disabilities.

One rule said that there was a list of rides on which a person with a disability could not ride without being accompanied by a "responsible adult," such being defined as any person over four feet tall. By that definition, Tina was a "responsible adult," and so, according to that same definition, was I. However, ValleyFair clearly didn't see things my way.

According to its rules, because I was blind, I was "required" to be accompanied by someone who could see whenever I went on many of its rides. The roller coaster and the corkscrew, two rides which I enjoyed immensely, were on the list of such rides. I was told that the rules were in place for reasons of "safety." After all, ValleyFair did not want a blind person riding something which might cause undue fear or trepidation.

It took me a couple of months to decide what to do. I am not a litigious person by nature. I don't go around suing people at the slightest provocation. However, ValleyFair's rule, requiring me to sit with a "responsible adult" who, by the park's own definition could be my sighted daughter, was something which I could not let stand.

I wanted ValleyFair to understand that blind parents take care of their sighted children—not the reverse. I wanted my daughter to understand that the problem we had with the roller coaster resulted from ignorance and lack of understanding. Most of all, I wanted to make things right for other blind people who might want to visit

ValleyFair. So, I decided that the only way to handle the problem was to file a charge of discrimination against ValleyFair with the Minnesota Human Rights Commission.

The details of the struggle which I and my friends in the National Federation of the Blind undertook with ValleyFair are not important. Suffice it to say that it took us five years for ValleyFair to eliminate its discriminatory rules, but eliminate them it did!

Today, blind people can visit ValleyFair and ride in peace. We don't have to visit Guest Relations to learn what attractions we are permitted to ride, and we can ride without having to be accompanied by a sighted person over four feet tall. Perhaps of more personal significance to me, my daughter, Tina, is proud of her father who, in her own words, "beat the pants off of ValleyFair!"

This is a battle which should not have had to be fought. If ValleyFair officials had learned about the capabilities of blind people before they developed the park's safety policies, they would never have created a rule requiring us to sit with a sighted person for many of its rides. If ValleyFair officials had talked the matter over with blind people themselves, its safety rules would have been more in keeping with reality.

THE BEST I HAVE
TO OFFER

by Mark A. Riccobono

Mark Riccobono is one of the young leaders in the National Federation of the Blind. Although he is only now in his early twenties, he is already president of our state organization in Wisconsin. His story is one which is repeated with unfortunate frequency:

A young child has poor vision. Teachers try to be kind and understanding. The eyesight gets worse or fails totally. Everyone tries to find a way to make do—just to get by. Especially if the child has a good mind, it is easy to pretend that he is doing "well enough." But no real effort is ever made to bring forth from that child the best he has to offer.

This is precisely the path Mark's life followed until he found the Federation through our scholarship program. Then it all changed. Here is what he has to say:

I have been legally blind since about age five from glaucoma. As a child I attended school very close to my home. I did everything else my friends did and learned at the same pace. In third grade, I began using large print books. This was my earliest hint of my blindness.

I continued for a long time doing all the things that others did. I was an active Boy Scout and even played on the softball team. I don't remember seeing the ball that well. Someone would stand in the outfield with me and tell me where the ball was. I was not headed for the majors, but I had fun with my friends and won some trophies.

As the years passed and my residual vision slowly deteriorated, I began to notice things I could not do, or at least I did not know how to do them, with poor eyesight. And

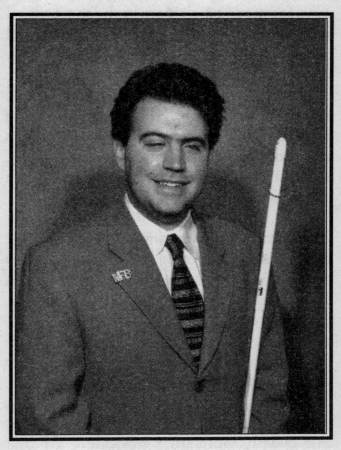

Mark Riccobono

some teachers did not challenge me and find ways for me to participate in the more visual activities. In certain areas I began to fall behind simply from not fully participating.

Nonetheless, I was good at many things, and learned others by listening and using what vision I had. For example, I always enjoyed math and was good with numbers. I could easily conceptualize it and work things out.

Reading, however, was not something I particularly enjoyed. Trying to focus my eyes on print was a burden and seemed, in the mind of a young boy with lots of energy, pointless.

Teachers exempted me from having to practice spelling words that were on the board because I could not read them. At other times, I would team up with a student in a class to work on a worksheet. By that time, I had gotten used to sliding by on these things and would sit passively while my friend, with careless haste, would do most of the work.

With idle time, I did become quite an expert in table football—a typical game to amuse a young person, which involved a piece of paper folded into a triangle. All of this left me idle with many thoughts and much energy not cultivated into learning and expanded knowledge.

I was the only blind student at both my elementary and middle school. An itinerant teacher from the public school vision program would come to see me once in a while to make sure I was getting along sufficiently. I was, but meeting the sufficiency standard was far below what, with the proper skills of blindness, I could have done.

I worked hard and my parents helped by reading to me and making sure I completed assignments. I was "successful."

I received good grades, participated in school activities, and had many friends. But no great effort was made to tap all of my abilities by telling me about resources available to the blind or introducing me to blind adult role models.

I never even knew another blind person until I reached high school. I chose the high school I did because it offered a specialized curriculum in business. To my benefit it also turned out that this school had a resource room for the visually impaired. It included computers equipped with speech and enlargement capabilities, a closed-circuit television for enlarging print materials, and a variety of other helpful tools.

This was the first time in my life I had ever gotten to know another blind person and, not to mention, become familiar with books on tape.

Even as I was introduced to these tools which would complement and help strengthen my abilities, I was still not as productive and independent as I should have been. In addition, I did not really think of myself as blind. I had a "visual impairment," whatever that meant. "I guess I am just unique," I thought without any real consideration about my attitudes or what impact this might have on my future.

I could have learned Braille there, but the attitude was passive and the benefits of using it were never stressed. I did not think it was worth my time. A tough curriculum was more important. Furthermore, no one offered this option to me in the summer when I had plenty of spare time.

In the meantime, my vision continued to deteriorate. I lost vision in my left eye completely in the same year I entered high school. Yet, with much assistance I continued to succeed. I strained to read print when I did not have tapes to depend on and became very dependent on memorizing because reading my notes was too difficult.

I would leave class and go to the resource room to work on assignments, removing myself from the camaraderie of my peers, which, for a teenager, is quite a sacrifice. I gave up much of my high school social life to complete work I could have done much more effectively had I known Braille and other skills of blindness.

Even so, I was very successful in high school. I received many awards and honors and was accepted to the University of Wisconsin. For the first two years of college much of the same trend continued. I used a short white cane from time to time, but it was more to look competent around college coeds than it was to travel safely and effectively.

In some classes, I used note takers who would give me copies of their notes because I could not effectively take and read my own. And, most damaging of all, I continued to struggle with my negative attitude about what blind people could really achieve and how I would ever accomplish my more lofty goals.

That is how things were until I won a scholarship from the National Federation of the Blind of Wisconsin and attended the National Convention in Anaheim, California. It was through the warm people I met and their positive attitudes that I finally began to realize the abilities I had hidden away and the tools that I needed to cultivate them.

I saw people using Braille effectively to take notes and share information. People walked confidently with long white canes so they could be independent and contribute all that they had to the convention.

Shortly after that convention, I began using a cane every day and learned Braille. I now travel confidently and safely. I can take notes which I can actually refer to later. I can carry reading material in Braille and spend all those little empty spaces of time, on buses and such, reading and studying.

The National Federation of the Blind helped me to use some of that extra ability I did not use because I did not have the proper tools. Now, I try to help other blind people realize the extent of their abilities through my work with the National Federation of the Blind. There are many young blind people out there who are in the same shoes I was in years ago. I want them to find and cultivate their abilities and use the most effective tools as early as possible, and I know the rest of the members of the organization feel the same.

When a sighted child shows some ability he or she is challenged and given greater opportunities to improve but, all too often, people are happy just to see a blind child achieve a minimal level of success.

I have come to the conclusion that untapped "ability" is our most abundant and underutilized resource. When we properly cultivate it and have a variety of tools we know how to use, sharpened ability begets ability. Booker T. Washington once said, "The world cares very little about what a man or woman knows. It is what the man or woman is able to do that counts."

This is what the National Federation of the Blind means when it stresses the importance of proper training in the skills of blindness, and it encourages blind people to work hard and dream big. I was always quite "successful," but with the "can do" attitude of the Federation and the skills of blindness I have developed, my success is now truly the best I have to offer.

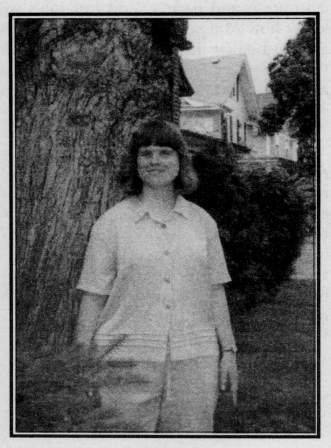

Kathy McGillivray

TAKING OUT THE GARBAGE

by Kathy McGillivray

Kathy McGillivray is a leader in the National Federation of the Blind of Minnesota. Her story here is about one of the most basic of household tasks—taking out the garbage. But, of course, it is about more than that.

Garbage comes in different forms. There is the kind you fill the trash can with and the kind you fill the mind with. As Kathy points out both kinds need to be cleaned out from time to time. Here is what she has to say:

The day had finally arrived. The last box had been hauled away from the apartment where I had lived for the past five years. I was excited. Finally I had a place of my own. No more paying rent. No more repeated calls to the caretaker to beg him to fix my sink. I was free at last.

I had just moved into my newly-purchased condominium and was happy to have more space and to live in a quieter neighborhood.

Overall, the move had gone relatively smoothly. In fact, this was the easiest move I could ever remember. Now that all ten of my volunteer moving crew had left, I decided it was time to take out some garbage.

We had already unpacked some of my boxes, and they were neatly stacked near the door. I decided it was time to get rid of them before the pile became too large.

I remember that, when I had first looked at the house, one of the other owners had warned me that the dumpster would be very difficult for me to find. She said I would probably need some help with it. She let me know about another blind person who had wandered several blocks looking for it. I told her that I appreciated her concern, but I would do just fine.

Hoisting my boxes onto my shoulder, I made my way down the back stairs and out to the parking lot. A sighted friend had informed me that I could go out and walk straight ahead for a few yards, take a left and go about twice as far again, and I would be at the dumpster.

I tried following these directions, but alas, no dumpster. I worked my way around several cars in the parking lot and searched for the dumpster but was unable to find it. Within a few minutes a woman came out and showed me where it was.

I thanked her politely but inwardly felt humiliated, frustrated, and even a bit angry. It was just not fair. I had just bought my own place, organized the move, and now I could not seem even to take out my own garbage.

A few days later I invited a friend to my house. My pile of boxes had grown rather large, and there were several bags of trash that needed to be taken out. I asked my friend for some assistance since there was so much to haul.

At this point there was a lot of snow in the back of the building, and many cars were parked there. My friend commented, "This is really going to be hard for you to find. There are really no landmarks; you just have to find your way through open space." She offered several suggestions for ways to locate the dumpster. I tried them later that week and was not very successful.

The reader of this account might be wondering why this was such a difficult task for me. The dumpsters are located across an alley, where many cars are parked, and the snow is not shoveled very well in the winter.

Several days later I asked the president of the condominium association whether it would be possible to move the dumpsters closer to the building. She said no.

Finally, I decided that enough was enough. I was going to find a way to locate these dumpsters, no matter how long it took. I grabbed my trash and headed outside.

This time I really made an effort to notice my surroundings and changes in the terrain as I moved closer to the dumpsters. Upon finding them, I took time to look around the whole area. I noticed that there was a garage within several feet of the dumpsters. I had also noted a fence and several trees along my path.

As I returned to my house, I wondered why nobody had pointed out these environmental cues to me, especially the garage. In a way I was glad they hadn't because it gave me the opportunity to discover them on my own.

By now, as you can probably guess, taking out the trash at my new place is a routine task, and I don't even think about it. While this was a relatively small incident in my life, it made me think about some garbage we blind people can collect in our attitudes if we are not careful.

One of the biggest pieces of garbage we can collect is the idea that sighted people have more information about the environment than blind people do and that they know best what we can do and how we should do it.

While sighted people can provide valuable information, they do not necessarily have all the information. As members of the National Federation of the Blind know, blind people are often the best teachers of other blind people.

A second piece of garbage we need to take out of our lives is excessive anger and frustration. Whether we are blind or sighted, if we are honest with ourselves, we all experience frustration in our lives to one degree or another.

Anger and frustration can be our friends if they move us to action. They can sound an alarm that calls us to wake up and make a change in our lives. At a certain level the National Federation of the Blind came into existence because of positive anger. Our early leaders were angry about the lack of opportunities for blind people and the negative stereotypes society often has about us, so they did something about it.

On the other hand, anger becomes an enemy when it paralyzes us and saps us of the creative energy we need to solve problems in our lives.

The third piece of garbage that needs to be disposed of is plain, old-fashioned laziness. If you're like me, you prefer things to be easy rather than hard. Unfortunately, much of life is not easy.

I think we all know several blind people who would rather have things done for them than learn the alternative techniques that would enable them to do things themselves. I fear that this attitude will not pay off in the end.

Just as I found a way to get my trash to the dumpster, all of us need to find ways to get rid of the garbage that collects in our lives. Through the work of the National Federation of the Blind, we can recognize that garbage and put it where it belongs.

LITTLE THINGS DO COUNT

by Patricia Maurer

Children are curious about blindness and are much less hesitant than are adults to ask questions about the things they really want to know. My wife, Patricia, frequently speaks to school children about how blind people do this and that—the little things of life. Here is her report of one such encounter:

I was in such a rush that morning. The kids got up late and would not get ready for school quickly. I didn't have the right change for their school lunches. They didn't want anything for breakfast and were both crabby in the car on the way to school.

My secretary was driving, and we were headed for a school to talk with fourth graders about how it is that blind people live their lives. Considering the frame of mind I was in, I remember thinking that it would have been much better that day if I could have gone back home for another cup of coffee or maybe to go back to bed.

When I got to the classroom, I was greeted by the teacher. She seemed to appreciate my coming very much. She said that the children had been reading a story about a blind woman and how she raised her daughter. She said that she thought I could answer some of the children's questions. She said that she didn't know the answers and didn't want to give the children wrong information.

I stood before the class. I used to teach elementary school. (I was blind then, too.) I enjoyed working with the children then, and I could see I was going to enjoy this class, too. I talked with the kids about Braille and showed them a book in Braille. I showed them a book called "The Boy Who Thought He Was A Dog." This book was in print, and the Braille had been added. I explained

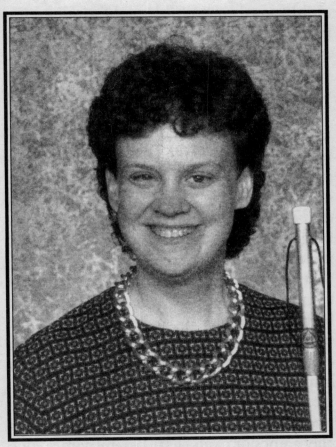

Patricia Maurer

that a blind parent could read to a sighted child or a blind child could read with a parent who could see. I had a Braille watch and a deck of Brailled playing cards. The children had to take a look at all of these things, and then they had questions.

One of the children asked how blind people can tell money apart. I explained how coins such as nickels, pennies, dimes, and quarters are easy to tell apart. They all are different sizes, and quarters and dimes have ridges around them, while pennies and nickels are smooth. There are many ways that paper money—like one, five, ten, or twenty-dollar bills—can be identified. Some blind people like to keep different bills in separate places in their wallets. The most common way to distinguish paper money is to fold the bills in different ways.

One of the boys asked if blind people can play games or cards. I said many games such as Scrabble can be played with Braille letters and a board with raised or tactile squares.

Backgammon boards can also be tactile and so can boards for chess or checkers. Pieces can be made of different textures, shapes, and colors to tell them apart, or a small piece of tape can be put on one set.

Monopoly cards can be Brailled, and the board can also be Brailled or marked. Yahtzee and other games using dice are easy if you use dice with dots that you can feel and count. Not all games have to be made especially for the blind. Many games and toys that you buy at the store are easy and fun for the blind. Sometimes you can use your imagination to think of ways that a blind person can use the same things as a sighted person.

One little girl noticed that my clothes matched, and she wondered how I knew what colors I was wearing. I said that most articles of clothing will have at least one distinct way of identifying them by feel. They will have different buttons or snaps or bows or ties or the fabric or texture will be different. Some dresses or skirts will have belts or elastic at the waist or different kinds of pockets. You might know that the red shirt is the one with the funny-shaped buttons, or the blue pants are the ones with no pockets. You can tell that the blouse with the fuzzy collar is green and is the one that matches the green pants with the belt that feels like rope. In this way, blind people can tell their clothes apart by touch, and they can tell what clothes match each other.

Sometimes, however, there may be more than one shirt or blouse that feels alike; men's ties can feel alike also. For these times, some blind people like to mark their clothes in a special way. There are tags that are meant for sewing in Braille labels, or a safety pin can be used to identify that this is a black pair of jeans.

Some people sew a button to the tag of a blue suit and cut out a corner of the tag on a gray suit. Some people make a list of the suits, shirts, ties, and other clothes that feel alike and match them with each other using Braille numbers and letters attached to each piece of clothing.

As I talked to the children, I told them that my husband and I are both blind and that we share the grocery shopping and cooking. The kids wondered how we bought our groceries. I told the children that there are many kinds of food that can be identified by touch, such as fruits and vegetables, hot dogs, chicken, and other items.

But things like cans of soup, cereal boxes, canned vegetables, gallons of milk, ice cream containers, and other things may be hard to identify. Many blind people like to shop with a friend who will help to find things and can read the different brands and types. Or a blind person might use a store employee who can help find the groceries.

We talked of many other things, and one of the final questions was how it feels to be blind. I said that when you are newly blind, in the beginning it can feel frustrating or scary. This is because you have not learned how to do things for yourself as a blind person. But once you learn the skills that blind people use, you no longer feel that way. Blind people do the same things as sighted people. We go to school or work, and we do the things that we need to do. We do this naturally, without even thinking about being blind. The blindness becomes just another part of who we are, and what we are like.

Time ran out before the questions were all answered. The teacher said that the children would be writing to me. She gave me a gift. It was a container of fudge, which she had made to thank me for coming.

The time I spent with the children that day and the letters which I received from them later made me think. We are all so busy with our jobs and our families that we sometimes do not realize that it is the little things that count.

A One-Way Trip to
St. Cloud

by Brad Hodges

Brad Hodges is a long-time leader in the National Federation of the Blind. Having lived in the Midwest most of his life, he recently accepted a position at the International Braille and Technology Center for the Blind in Baltimore, Maryland. Brad's new job requires him to be creative and resourceful. But this is not a problem for him. He's been at it a long time as this story from his college days demonstrates. Here is what he has to say:

Selecting a college is a task in which the student and his or her family consider many factors and make many decisions. As I approached my graduation from high school in the mid-1970's I faced the daunting task of choosing from among many excellent private colleges.

After much consideration, trips to prospective schools, and discussion I chose St. John's University located in Collegeville, Minnesota.

St. John's is located in the pine forest of central Minnesota. The natural environment is a constant presence for those who visit the campus and especially for those of us who lived there. Two lakes and miles of walking paths provided many hours of enjoyment amid the natural beauty of the woods.

Because the campus was not near any town, the university offered bus service to the College of Saint Benedict, St. John's sister institution, in nearby St. Joseph, Minnesota. Although shopping was available in St. Joseph, St. Cloud, a twelve-mile trip from St. John's, was where the real action was.

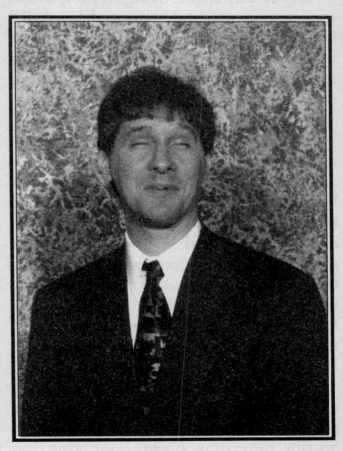

Brad Hodges

Very shortly after arriving on campus and settling into my freshman residence hall I began to consider exactly what technique would be best in order to arrange for a predictable and sufficient supply of transportation to St. Cloud.

I am the eldest of three sons. My parents taught all of their boys many valuable lessons and saw to it that we left home with the knowledge and skills required to survive in the adult world. In my mother's opinion one of the essential skills which everyone must be able to perform is that of ironing clothes. For this reason I packed my own ironing board and shiny new Hamilton Beach iron with the other necessities of student life.

In the late 1970's formal dances and other social activities were still very much alive and part of the social calendar at St. John's. Naturally every guy on my floor wanted to look his very best, so as to impress his date for the evening.

Interestingly, I was the only guy on my floor who had an iron, ironing board, and the knowledge and skill to use them.

As you can imagine, my buddies soon discovered this and began asking me to press their shirts for these formal occasions. I thought to myself, well, what is the value of a pressed shirt to these guys? The answer soon emerged: it's worth a one-way trip to or from St. Cloud.

When the Saturday of the next formal occasion arrived I let it be known that if you had your laundered shirt to my room by 4:00 p.m. you would have it back by 6:00. In exchange for which you would provide me a one-way trip to or from St. Cloud.

This bartering was acceptable to all those who had cars and wanted to look good on Saturday night. As a result I never went without transportation to or from St. Cloud.

As a blind student I wanted to enjoy the many valuable features of St. John's. At the same time I needed an alternative technique to address the dilemma of living in a rural setting and not having independent access to my own car. My mother's insistence that her boys had the knowledge and skills to maintain their clothes proved to be a double blessing.

You can help us spread the word...

...about our Braille Readers Are Leaders contest for blind schoolchildren, a project which encourages blind children to achieve literacy through Braille.

...about our scholarships for deserving blind college students.

...about Job Opportunities for the Blind, a program that matches capable blind people with employers who need their skills.

...about where to turn for accurate information about blindness and the abilities of the blind.

Most importantly, you can help us by sharing what you've learned about blindness in these pages with your family and friends. If you know anyone who needs assistance with the problems of blindness, please write:

Marc Maurer, President
National Federation of the Blind
1800 Johnson Street, Suite 300
Baltimore, Maryland 21230-4998

Other Ways You Can Help the National Federation of the Blind

Write to us for tax-saving information on bequests and planned giving programs.

OR

Include the following language in your will:

"I give, devise, and bequeath unto National Federation of the Blind, 1800 Johnson Street, Suite 300, Baltimore, Maryland 21230, a District of Columbia nonprofit corporation, the sum of $_____ (or "___ percent of my net estate" or "The following stocks and bonds:_____") to be used for its worthy purposes on behalf of blind persons."

Your Contributions Are Tax-deductible